Aging Is A Family Affair

Planning the Care of Elderly Loved Ones

by Doug Manning

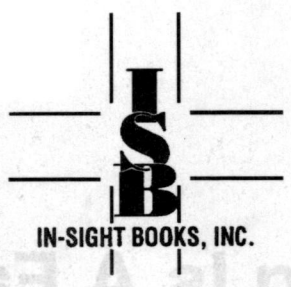

In-Sight Books

Copyright©1998 by In-Sight Books, Inc.
P. O. Box 42467
Oklahoma City, Oklahoma 73123
1-800-658-9262

All rights reserved. No part of this book may be reproduced in any form or by any means without prior written permission of the publisher, excepting brief quotes used in connection with reviews, written specifically for inclusion in a magazine or newspaper.

Manufactured in the United States of America

ISBN 1-892785-27-7

Dedication

To

Joe Hoyle
1924-1998
Uncle, Friend, "Roadie", Christian Gentleman

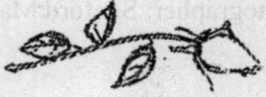

Cover Photo

Special thanks to:
Audrey Dragg
Don Dragg
Kim Dragg
Jennifer Dragg
Matthew Dragg
Morgan Dragg

Photographer: Sanford Mauldin

Table of Contents

The Family Decision — 7
    Thinking the Unthinkable — 8
    The Meeting No One Wants to Have — 12
    Many Are Called—You Are Chosen — 14
    Nice Ways to Say It — 18
    The Meeting—Oh! The Dreaded Meeting — 19
    Wait A Minute, You Mean The Parents Are There Too? — 21
    The Magic of Communication — 24
    A Bill of Rights for the Caregiver — 28

The Agenda — 33
    Get Thee to a Lawyer — 34
    What About the Money? — 36
    Discovering the Levels of Care — 41
    When Do We Make the Decision? — 48
    End of Life Decisions — 51

The Care Process — 55
    Make Friends With the Physician — 56
    No One Wants to Spy On Their Own Parents — 59
    If Care is Needed — 63
    How to Select a Care Facility — 66
    Planning the Move — 70
    Building Communication — 75
    The Unblessed Child — 84
    Gifts That Communicate — 87
    Taking Care of You — 92

The Tool Chest 97
　Checklist for Moving a Loved One
　　Into Your Home 101
　Checklist for Initial Visit to a Care Facility 103
　Selecting a Care Facility 105
　Admission to A Nursing Home 109
　Medicaid Information 111
　Alternative Methods of Financing 112

Section One
The Family Decision

Chapter One

Thinking About the Unthinkable

No one knows they are old. I have asked many people what it feels like to be old and I get the same quizzical look every time. No one knows they are. Athletes don't know when to retire because they don't know they have lost a step or some reaction time. It still feels the same and they have no idea they have aged. Everyone thinks they are about twenty years younger than they really are. I think I am forty-five. I used to think I was thirty-five until I was walking as fast as I could through an airport. It felt like it did when I was twenty-five. The wind was whipping through my hair. I was moving with the same old grace and speed, and little old ladies were passing me. I became forty-five that day.

My father often visited the residents of a nursing home. Every time he went he would announce that he was going to go visit the "old folks in the nursing home." He was eighty-five at the time. Only three people in the home were as old as he was, but he didn't know it. He thought he was young.

We not only don't realize we are getting old—we have no idea that we will ever grow any older. I have conducted seminars on elder care decisions for fifteen years, and yet I personally have no concept that I will ever need any of my advice. I don't think I'll ever need to be cared for. I certainly won't need my children involved in any long-term care decisions. My speech is fine for seminars but it has nothing to do with me or my wife. We are much too young to even give it a thought.

I also thought my parents and my in-laws would never get old. They weren't going to need any outside care. If they did get old and needed help they could just move in with me. I promised them over and over that they would never live in a nursing home. My parents said they would rather die than go to a nursing home and I said, "Not to worry, it will never happen."

My mother-in-law died in a nursing home. My father died in a nursing home. My mother died in an assisted living center. Needless to say I have had to face some radical changes in my thinking. I had to face a rather rude awakening in my world. Now my family needs to face this same kind of awakening. Like it or not, want to think about it or not, ready or not, my family needs to begin thinking through the realities we may face a long time before we are ready to do so.

When I was in my forties an old man said, "If you don't die you're going to get old." I thought, "Now that is a profound statement if I ever heard one. Everyone knows that." But I **didn't** know that, and it **was** a profound statement. If we don't die we will get old, and, like it or not, I must face the issues that come with getting old. Like it or not, I need to get my head out of the sand and think about these issues now, in advance of the day.

I may need care. I cannot imagine that ever happening, but I could not imagine it happening to my parents either.

My family may have to go through placing me in some kind of care facility. They might have to do so against my will.

My wife might have to go through the agony of going against her promise to care for me for better or worse until death do us part.

I might have to face that same decision with my wife whom I have loved through forty-five years of marriage.

We need to think about these things and we need to prepare to do so long before the need arises. Most long-term care decisions are made on the spur of the moment. The doctor says our loved one must leave the hospital and they can no longer live at home. At that point the family has about twenty-four hours to find a solution to the problem. The urgency of the situation leaves very little time to really compare facilities. There is no time for family planning. There is not enough time to involve family members who cannot be present when the decisions must be made.

Even if we luck out and find a great facility, many unresolved issues remain. This sets the stage for the possibility of deep divisions in the family. Far too many loose ends remain dangling which become harder and harder to tie down after the decision has already been made.

If a family is ever going to have a fight it will probably happen over the issue of how to care for aging loved ones. I know of many wonderful families who have been ripped apart by this controversy and no longer speak to each other. I have witnessed many court fights over how the money was spent. Most of this turmoil could have been avoided if they had known how to face these issues before there was a crisis. Being forced to make decisions under the stress of too little time sets the stage for most of the family struggles.

The best advice I can give is for the family to begin discussing these issues long before care is needed. A family meeting should be organized for this purpose. The best time to have such a meeting is when most of the family's response is, "Why are we doing this now?"

Chapter 2

The Meeting No One Wants to Have

When I start talking about having a family meeting to discuss the long-term care of our loved ones the audiences visibly stiffen up. I see fear on almost every face. We are afraid to talk to our families. No one wants to confront parents and siblings. We fear things will get out of hand and we will never get them resolved. Family members are always harder to talk to than anyone else. They mean too much to us for us to take the risk. Since they will be a part of our lives forever, it is difficult to be open and vulnerable to them. As a minister, I have talked with many terminally ill people. I have learned to be comfortable talking with them about their dying. When my brother was dying, I made three trips to talk with him. Each time I sat on his bed and never said a word. We were brothers and it was too close.

We want all of these issues to just work themselves out on their own. We want to be able to simply hint or look hurt and have the rest of the family able to read our minds.

At a recent conference a minister told about his in-laws moving into his house. He said, "They are wonderful people and are more than welcome in our home. They have their own private area of the house but they seem to want to spend all of their time with us. How can I let them know that we need our space and our private time?" I said, "And the rest of your sentence is how can we do that without having to say anything to them, right?" He said "Right."

The problem is we can't convey these hard messages without saying something. It may hurt at the time, but hurting now is much better than allowing unspoken issues to become a constant irritant that drives a family apart. Unspoken feelings do not disappear, they tend to fester and grow into major issues and grudges. You will hear me say this again and again, the only way to avoid misunderstanding is to have an understanding. The only way to have an understanding is to get together and hear the feelings and thoughts of each member of the family.

It's like the guy who was going to cut off the dog's tail. He could not stand to do it all at once so he cut it off a little at a time. Confrontation is painful and frightening, but if we choose to avoid all conflict we end up dealing with each step and issue as a separate battle. The pain and anger increase with each battle.

Chapter 3

Many Are Called—You Are Chosen

One member of the family will usually become the primary caregiver. This can happen because one member lives closer to the parents than all of the others. Or, it may be that this member has just always been the one everyone depended on for care. These chosen ones may be the strongest ones in their family, or, in many cases, they are the ones most easily manipulated by other family members.

If the person happens to be a nurse or engaged in some other form of health care, they are automatically elected for the care task in the family. One way or the other, the family will try to hang it on one member of the family. I call this phenomenon "many are called—**you are chosen.**"

When one member becomes the primary caregiver, the rest of the family is free to sit back and second-guess every decision the person makes. I hear unbelievable stories from such caregivers. Not only do they give the care with very little help or support, they labor under constant criticism and complaint from the rest of the family.

Therefore, the person most likely to be the primary caregiver must be the one to call the family meeting. No one else will take the initiative and why would they? Otherwise the situation remains set up exactly like the rest of the family wants it to be. If the primary caregiver allows this at the beginning of the process, then the situation cements and they are locked into the job. They can expect very little help and even less sympathy for their commitment and service.

Typically, at this point, the response is, "You don't know my family. There is no way they will come to such a meeting." The truth is your family is probably not all that different. All families have members who react differently when faced with a problem. Some will be in total denial. They can't see anything wrong with the loved ones no matter what their condition may be. They will argue against the need for the meeting. Other members of the family will be in total panic, "Mother is dying and **you** are not doing anything about it. Her doctor is a quack and the facilities here are inadequate." Every family will have some realist in the group who can give some stability to the meeting. The realist must lead the way both in the meeting and probably in the long-term care to follow.

There may be members of the family who do not want to come to the meeting. When I tell groups the answer to this is to say, "You either attend the meeting or I am going to mail Mother to you", they think I am joking, but I'm not.

Divisions may already exist in some families. It is not uncommon for some members of the family to have isolated themselves from the family unit. Some may not have spoken to other members of the family for years. Splits can occur even in the finest of families. When this is true the chances are they will not attend the meeting no matter how much effort is made. In those cases the meeting should go on without them present. Every effort to include them should still be made. Sometimes an event like this can jar a family member into realizing that life is passing and that it is time to get beyond old grudges. Even if they refuse, at least they were given the chance to participate and can't use their exclusion as further fodder for their anger or hurt.

Often a spouse must call the meeting. When a spouse is beginning to fail, a wise individual will ask the family to talk about the future. Facing the long-term care of a spouse is one of the most difficult things a person can experience. A wife feels like she is going against every sinew in her body. She promised to love "till death do us part" and now she is forsaking her love in his time of need. The husband may have the greatest struggle of all. He is the "fixer" the one who takes care of things. To him this means admitting defeat.

I encourage spouses to call the meeting even though they dread it like the plague. As the conditions deteriorate they will need the support of the children. One of the great needs we have in caregiving is an objective view. The children's view might not be very objective, but it will certainly be more so than that of a spouse. And, if the time comes when the loved one needs to become a resident of some care facility, the children need to be there to give the spouse a push. My mother could never have made the decision about my father without the push from my brother and me.

Even only children need to have a family meeting. An only child must face all of these decisions with very little outside help and, believe me, they have never been as alone as they will be during the time of long-term care decisions. An only child needs to have the family meeting while one or both parents are alive. It will be a great help to know what the parents' feelings are and, if possible, to have their support. An only child may also enlist the aid of some selected aunts, uncles or cousins. If I were an only child I would try to make a friend of someone who is also facing long-term care decisions, or one who has already gone through the process may be even more help.

No one should try to face these issues alone. Yet many primary caregivers do face it alone. Many times they are alone, even though they have family who could help, because the family was allowed to hang all of the cares on that person. The purpose and aim of this book is finding relief for lonely caregivers.

Chapter 4

Nice Ways to Say It

Since communicating with family members is difficult, maybe a sample letter will help.

> Dear_____
>
> The older I get the more my family means to me. I guess when we are young we take it all for granted. We may not realize the importance of the people we call family or the place we call home. Then as life slips by, and so many other things seem to be fleeting, we suddenly realize how great it is to have the rock of a family to depend upon.
>
> In the years ahead, as our parents grow older, our family will be facing some tough questions. Caring for elderly loved ones requires decisions that none of us should make alone. The only way to avoid misunderstanding is to have an understanding. I do not want misunderstandings to drive wedges in our family and the only way I know to avoid such a thing is to meet and fully discuss the issues we will face in the future.
>
> I hope all of us can get together this summer, (or give a set date), for a time of open discussion about how we will handle the issues of the future. We need to know how each one of us thinks and feels about these concerns.
>
> Love,

Chapter 5

The Meeting—Oh! The Dreaded Meeting

If you are the primary caregiver, it is very important that you follow some guidelines in the meeting. You will probably be in charge, but you need to make everyone else talk first. Don't get caught in the trap of saying what you think and then asking for their opinions. Ask each person to express how they see the future and how they see the options that are available. Don't let there be any spectators. Spectators become critics.

We need to understand the family dynamics that will be present in most meetings. Each person there will have a different relationship to the parents. Each person there will respond to the needs of the parents in their own manner.

Some may have feelings of inferiority and think they have never been accepted by the family. Some may feel as if they have never been able to live up to their parents' expectations and are somehow not as loved as the other children. Some may be reacting to years of too much parental control. These folks are what I call the "unblessed children." We will talk about their situation in more detail in a later chapter.

All we need to realize right now is that some members of the family will come to the meeting carrying various kinds of baggage and will react from a position governed by that baggage.

Some may be there who carry a heavy load of anger and unfinished agendas about the parents. It will be hard for them to be objective and focused in their discussion. They may need to spend some time talking about the past. These folks simply need to be heard. Arguing with them or explaining their pain away will only make matters worse.

Others may be there who have distanced themselves both by geography and emotions. They will find it hard to get into the discussion with any emotional involvement at all. They will appear cold to the rest of the group but that is where they are and they are the only ones who can change their feelings.

All this means is that each group will be made up of different people with different relationships and different needs. Each one must be allowed to struggle in their own way. Each one must have the right to decide how much they share. Those who cry do not necessarily care more than those who do not. If this is a time of great acceptance then this can be a time of great healing.

The parents themselves need special understanding. They may feel invaded against their will. They may feel someone is taking control over their lives. They may not be ready to even think about long-term care. It is vital that their concerns be very carefully heard.

Chapter 6

Wait A Minute, You Mean the Parents Are There Too?

There may be times when the children need to have a preliminary meeting to get their thinking coordinated and on the same page. Those families who are dealing with Alzheimer's or other forms of dementia will need to have meetings without the loved one present. But, as a general rule, the whole family needs to be involved in this meeting. It does make the meeting a lot scarier. But think of how you would feel if you were old and a meeting was called to discuss your future. If the meeting was about me I'd want to be there.

Far too often we make decisions about our parents without talking to them, and then wonder why they resent what we decided. At almost every conference I hear, "Why won't they listen to me? They can't take care of themselves anymore and I have told them and told them but they will not listen." I always ask, "Were they involved in the decision? Did anyone listen to what they wanted? Did anyone listen to why they are so adamant about taking care of themselves?"

We began this plan book by talking about the fact that no one knows they are old. It takes time and a lot of support before we can come to grips with our true condition. Just having someone say we are old does not mean we believe it. Even when the facts are undeniable we can still believe it in our heads and not believe it at all in our emotions.

This kind of talking to our parents feels strange and difficult. The roles seem reversed. We aren't comfortable and neither are they. We have spent our lives trying to avoid parental anger, and suddenly we are confronting it face to face. "What if they get mad? What if they hate me the rest of their lives?"

Feeling guilty makes the problem even worse. Most of us were raised feeling a great deal of guilt in our relationship with our parents. Parents often use guilt as a tool to keep us in line. When we must confront them about these unpleasant subjects all of the old guilt tapes in our minds begin playing at the same time and we panic. Our heart rate jumps, our blood pressure soars, and we have an overwhelming urge to run away and hide. We want to change the subject. We want to only talk about pleasant things.

Some folks react to this with anger. They get mad at their parents. These are the people who scream out in frustration at the conferences. Others react by avoiding the whole issue. They simply change the subject and hope it all works out. There are thousands of folks living in very bad situations because their children can't stand to confront the parents or challenge the situation.

If we can get past the initial fear and guilt. If we can let our parents get past the initial flash of anger and resentment, we can communicate. Believe it or not, communication can happen even with **your** parent who may be different from any other parent on earth. Not only is it possible to communicate—I think we must.

Chapter 7

The Magic of Communication

Decisions about the care of our aging loved ones forces us to try to communicate under as much stress and emotional turmoil as we will ever face. Having a family meeting will not make it easy to communicate. The meeting is tough but in the long run well worth the effort. Whether or not we have a family meeting, we still face the issue of communicating about tough decisions no one wants to make.

Even though the family members may have differing opinions, and the parents may be in the shock stage of grief, communication is still possible. May I offer you some rather magical rules for communicating under stress?

1. Most of the time people just want to be heard and understood. We all need the chance to explain how we feel about what is happening to us. After we have been heard we can move on. If we feel ignored and are made to feel insignificant, we react negatively. If ignored long enough the issue becomes an obsession to us and we cannot see beyond the obsession.

The meeting needs to start by carefully listening to each person's thoughts and feelings. We may not agree. Matter of fact we may disagree completely, but this is not the time to say so. There will be plenty of time later. Now is the time for learning where folks are and letting them experience the joy of being heard. Timing is everything in communication. It is not what we say nor how we say it, it is when we say it that matters. If someone knows we have heard them, then we can say almost anything and not be offensive. If they do not feel as though they have been heard, then anything we say can be offensive.

One of the most powerful communication statements is, "May I tell you what I am hearing you say?" That says I have heard you and what you have to say is so important to me that I want to be sure I get it right. Try that on the most difficult family member and watch the belligerence mellow out.

2. You can't change the way people feel by changing the way they think. Feelings do not necessarily follow thoughts. How many times have you heard someone say. "I know that is the truth but that is not how I feel about it." Feelings change when someone crawls into the feelings with us and understands what we feel. Somehow we no longer need to defend the feelings and can relax. Quite often the relaxation leads to a change in feelings.

3. Arguing will not change the way someone feels. Feelings change from inside out. Argument forces people to build walls of defense and fight change. If they are allowed to express what they feel, and are heard, they can let go of the defenses and change can happen. Often they do not know what they feel or why they feel the way they do. Talking not only lets us know where they are, but it can also let the person discover a great deal about themselves and their feelings. Discovery is the beginning of change.

We may have an overwhelming urge to argue, but if we can resist this impulse, amazing things can happen. It may come slowly and it will not always work, but the success rate of the listening ear is miles ahead of the pitiful results of argument.

4. Anger grows until someone is sorry. I waited a long time in a restaurant. The manager came in person to apologize and offered the meal without charge. I told him the wait was not that long and there was no need for him to not charge us for our meal. At another restaurant I observed someone complaining about the slow service. The manager argued with them and tried to justify the waiting time. The longer he talked, the madder they got. He never said he was sorry.

Often there will be members of the family who arrive at the meeting with their anger already boiling, or with a chip on their shoulder. If we listen and simply say we are sorry they feel the way they do or are sorry about whatever caused the feelings to be there, the anger can begin to dissipate. This may not always work, but it is certainly worth the try.

5. Focus on the needs and not the faults. I tell my marriage counseling clients to talk about their needs and not their partner's faults. Saying "I need a hug" is much better than saying "You never hug me" The latter comes across as an attack. In the family meeting we need to say, "Mother needs our support and presence," instead of, "Why don't you ever go see your mother?" Or maybe even worse, "I go see Mother every day and she cries because the rest of you are too busy to go see her."

6. Focus on solutions instead of problems. When folks are having to make decisions they do not want to make or take action they are not ready to take, they will have a reason why every solution offered will not work. That can be quite frustrating and create a great deal of confusion in the group. When someone starts explaining why everything mentioned will not work, a good approach is to say, "I know this is not the answer we all want but tell us what you think we should do? What do you see as the first step?" This puts the ball in their court. No argument. No accusations. Just a simple, "What, then, is your solution?" This may be a little mean, but it's effective.

Chapter 8
A Bill of Rights for the Caregiver

In most cases one of the family members will end up being the primary caregiver. Sometimes one child will combine with a parent in the care of the other parent and gradually become the caregiver to both. Sometimes two or more of the children will live close enough to share the care, but even in these cases one child evolves with most of the responsibility and decision making.

We have become a scattered society. In years past, if there were six children in the family, five of them would continue to live in the general area. In these times all six will have moved away. There is no longer a core group of family available to care for the aging. This has caused the necessity of long-term care facilities. It has also put a burden on one or two members in the family. These become the primary caregivers.

Far too often the rest of the family takes advantage of these caregivers.

Far too often the primary caregiver suffers in silence because the same kindness that causes them to be willing to care also makes them avoid confrontation.

Far too often the primary caregiver must also endure the criticisms and second-guessing of the absent family members.

Usually it will be evident who the primary caregivers will be by the time the family meeting is over. Before adjourning the meeting I think the family needs to make a list of caregiver rights and take a pledge to assure these rights are given in the right spirit. The list should include such things as:

1. **The Right to Rest** — Caregiving is emotionally and physically draining work. The caregiver needs frequent breaks. Most caregivers tend to over-do and will need more breaks than they are willing to take, so the family needs to organize themselves into a care watch for the caregiver. Insist on breaks.

They will also need at least an annual vacation. Both short breaks and longer vacations can be arranged by other members of the family taking over for a time. If no family member is available, nursing homes offer what is called respite care. Respite care means they will care for your loved one for a week or so at a time without their having to be fully admitted to the facility.

Many times the family needs to insist that the caregiver take advantage of such things as adult day care and other programs available in many communities. I am always amazed at how many of these programs go unused while a family member works themselves almost to death. The family should monitor the caregiver and help them not to become totally consumed by the care.

2. Don't Criticize Behind the Back of the Caregiver — I have had far too many caregivers weep as they told me how hard it is to not only care for a loved one but to bear the nitpicking and criticism of their siblings. If you have a criticism then go to the caregiver in person and use the magic words and the magic ears until there is an agreement reached.

I have told more than one caregiver who was being criticized over the expenses and how the books were being kept to simply mail the checkbook to the complaining party and refuse to take it back. Don't criticize unless you are willing to do the job yourself. If we would follow that simple rule a great deal of peace could break out in the family.

3. Be Sensitive to the Caregivers' Time and Expense — If a loved one becomes a resident of a facility, the home of the primary caregiver becomes the motel for the rest of the family when they come for a visit. When my mother-in-law and my father were in nursing homes, we became full time inn keepers. A constant stream of folks came to see the parents. There are expenses involved in feeding and housing that many people. Over time this can become quite draining. There is also a great consumption of time involved. The extra cost was not as much of a problem to me as the time lost from work and the loss of private time with my family.

When you go, be sure you are not an overload. When you go, don't expect to be fed every meal.

4. **You Are Not the Doctor** — Caregiving means making a whole lot of decisions we don't want to make. A constant stream of medical questions require answers. Too often we must answer these with a minimum of information. Caregiving is a process of doing your best and hoping it all works out. Then family members come to visit and question every thing that has been done medically. They attack the doctor as being incompetent. The caregiver is grilled about medical procedures. Confidence that was already shaky is destroyed. And then the family goes home. The caregiver is back to making decisions but with more fear than ever. Do I need to spell it out any clearer than that?

5. **Don't Forget to Say Thank You** — When my mother-in-law died, my wife's brother and sister insisted that my wife and I go on a trip paid for out of the estate. The trip was wonderful and needed. The thoughtfulness of the thank you felt even better than the trip.

Section Two
The Agenda

Chapter 9
Get Thee to a Lawyer

While the family is still together it is a good idea to have a visit with an attorney. There are now many attorneys who specialize in Elder Law. This would be a preferred choice but if one is not available most attorneys either have enough general knowledge or know how to find answers to meet the need.

This is the time to discuss, and possibly sign, a document called Advanced Directives. This is better known as A Living Will, but Advanced Directives are much more detailed than the old Living Will forms we once used. Modern medicine is both a blessing and a curse. We now live much longer, but dying is much harder to accomplish. If the loved ones do not want heroic measures done to resuscitate them, well written Advanced Directives are vital. Since these documents are becoming more detailed and explicit, it is best to have the services of an attorney who has the necessary legal information to make these as effective as possible.

Another needed document is a Durable Power Of Attorney For Health Care. This simply gives chosen family members the right to make health care choices in case a person is not coherent enough to make decisions.

It is a good idea to also have a Durable Power of Attorney for Finance issued as protection in case the loved one becomes incompetent to make financial decisions. The person given this power of attorney does not have to exercise the power until there is a need, but when there is a need it is too late to take this precaution. Strokes, accidents and Alzheimer's Disease often leave a family with no power over the finances without appearing in court. Signing this may make the loved one feel a loss of control, but, if they will think of the consequences, they may welcome the chance.

Chapter 10

What About the Money?

The lawyer or financial planner can also help the family make arrangements for dealing with financial matters. When my mother-in-law was in our care, we set ourselves up for a tremendous family fight. My wife's brother and sister are wonderful and trusting people so the fight did not happen. We transferred my mother-in-law's money into a joint account with my wife. If this is done it only takes one family member saying, "You did not spend the money right," and the fight is on. I can't tell you how many stories I hear such as, "I took care of my mother. My brothers did not help in any way and now they are suing me over the money."

We did not have a family fight, but we spent three years trying to explain the transactions to the Internal Revenue Service. Somehow they cannot fathom two people working out of the same account.

A lawyer, a financial planner, or a competent accountant can show the family methods for handling and reporting the finances to avoid disagreement. Hopefully a realistic picture of the cost will be presented to the family. Unless they have already experienced a situation of care they will probably not realize the expenses involved and may become disgruntled at the cost. This is another time when understanding is the only way to avoid misunderstanding.

Alternative Methods of Financing

Most people are surprised to learn that Medicare does not pay for long-term care. After a person on Medicare has been in the hospital for 3 days then Medicare will pay for 100 days of recovery time in a nursing home. Actually Medicare pays 100% of the first 20 days and 80% of the rest of the 100 days of care. If they go back to the hospital for another 3 days then they can qualify for another 100 days of care. To qualify for these periods of care the patient must be making progress toward recovery. Except for those situations Medicare does not pay.

Medicaid will cover the cost of long-term care for those patients who do not have other means of financial support. The rules for this coverage vary by state, but, in general, the person must have less than $2,000.00. If they have a house and a living spouse, the spouse can live in the house. If they live in a house alone the house must be sold and the money used up in care before Medicaid will begin to pay. Since the states set the amount of money they will pay, the nursing homes must limit the number of such patients they take. Naturally this means Medicaid beds are getting harder to find.

The family needs to do some long range planning if a person is going to qualify for Medicaid. Giving away assets at the last minute to qualify is not allowed. The Government can go back three years and look at gifts and asset transfers. Any moneys given in that period may need to be used in care before the person qualifies.

There was a time when Social Security payments would cover the cost of a long-term care facility. Like all other medical costs, the cost of long-term care has gone up considerably while the state reimbursements to nursing homes has been reduced. This makes long-term care cost more than Social Security or most retirement programs can cover. Some kind of supplemental income is necessary if a loved one is a resident of most long-term care facilities. This makes long term financial planning a necessity.

Even if the family is planning to supplement the cost of care, there needs to be clear understanding about how much, how long, when the payments will be made, and who will handle the funds. Too often we come to some kind of vague promise to "Help all I can," and in the process set the stage for some very hard feelings.

If the loved one has funds to supplement the retirement or Social Security, the need for planning still exists. How long will the funds last? How will they be dispersed? Who will help the loved one keep track of the bank account and check book? What kind of reports and information about the finances do the rest of the family want to receive? How often should these reports be submitted?

If the family is going to fight, it will probably be over the money. If there is a need for understanding anywhere it is in this area.

Recently, I have bumped into some alternate methods of financing long-term care that I did not know about. I am not recommending any of these, but thought they should be brought to the attention of folks who are looking for answers to the financial burden of long-term care.

Reverse Mortgages Most states have passed laws that make it possible for an aging loved one to make what is called a reverse mortgage on their house and use the money to live on or to provide long-term care for themselves. A loan against the equity of the home is issued. This is not like other loans because it does not require monthly payments. Payments or a lump sum is received by the home owner who can live in the home as long as they wish. When the person no longer lives in the home, the heirs can either sell the home and pay off the mortgage or pay off the mortgage and keep the home. Since these homes are backed by FHA and Fannie Mae the home owner will never owe more than the home is worth. An interview with a Reverse Mortgage company is included in the Tool Chest section.

Viatical Settlements This is a very new concept. If a loved one has a terminal or chronic illness, viatical companies will purchase the life insurance policies. The loved one receives a cash payment which is tax free and can be used for care in any way they please. The viatical company keeps the insurance in force and collects the death benefit at the proper time. See the Tool Chest for details.

Long-term care Insurance After caring for both of our parents, my wife and I bought a long-term insurance policy on ourselves. We are now covered no matter what kind of care we need in the future. Even though the cost of this insurance escalates with age, it is worth looking into for our aging loved ones. With the cost of care rising it may be economically feasible even for older loved ones. An interview with a long-term care insurance agent can be found in The Tool Chest.

Chapter 11

Discovering the Levels of Care

There was a time when the long-term care of a loved one was quite simple. When the parents got old they moved in with one of the children and lived there until they died. Nursing homes as we know them did not exist until the sixties. Before that time the only care outside of the home was some nice lady in town who loved old people and cared for them in her home. It is easy to look back at those days and wonder if we built nursing homes because we stopped loving our parents. Or to feel as if we do not love our parents as much as the past generations did.

Nursing facilities are the outgrowth of some major changes in our society and in the way we live. The fact that people now are living longer has forced us to find other sources of care. We aren't living longer because we stopped getting sick. We are living longer because we now live with diseases that once took our lives. Living with these diseases means we need much more care. We are now living beyond our children's ability to care for us. I promised my father he would never go to a nursing home. I kept my promise, but he outlived the promise. He needed more care than I could provide at home. There was a time when moving a loved one into our homes was less than a five year commitment. Now the care can last for as long as twenty years.

We have also become a scattered society. There is no longer a core group of family living in the old home town and available to care for the aging. Matter of fact it is almost rare when any of the children still live in the home town.

We have also become a society of two income families. There is no one at home during the day to give care.

Because of these changes, long-term care is no longer a simple decision. This makes it imperative that we look at all of the options and make our choices with as much information as possible.

Home Care

Even with the changes in our society, home care is still a viable option for many families. With the care available through home health agencies the care of a loved one at home is somewhat easier than before. Home health professionals provide help with administering medications, checking blood pressure, checking and changing the dressings on wounds and incisions, and, in some cases, help with bathing. Home health cannot provide day long nursing care in the home.

Many families can afford and can find nursing help to stay with loved ones around the clock. This care is, of course, quite expensive and hard to maintain, but it is one option.

Moving a loved one into the home of a family member is the most often chosen option of all. At least that is where the care starts. I moved my mother-in-law into my home and intended to care for her until she died. It did not work out like I expected but that is where the care started. If you are thinking of caring for a loved one in your home, read the information on that subject in the Tool Chest section of this book.

The Levels of Long-Term Care

There was a time when there was only one type of nursing home. The choices were limited and the decisions were simple. Now a whole continuum of care is available. The care is specialized to fit the actual condition of the loved one. This makes starting early even more important. We need time to evaluate the loved one and time to find the facility that fits their particular needs. The last thing a family wants to do is pay for more care than is needed. The loved one will be much happier in a place that specializes in the kind of care needed and where the residents are dealing with the same needs and limitations. They will do best in a place where they can understand and support each other. Some of the types of care now available are:

Retirement Living—The first level of care would be retirement facilities. These vary in type and cost. Many retirement communities are sponsored by nonprofit or religious groups and offer a full range of possibilities from retirement cottages to a dormitory arrangement. Most of these have certain rules to determine whether or not an individual is qualified for the center. Usually the person must be able to come to the meals without assistance. Some will not allow the use of wheel chairs or walkers in meeting this requirement.

Some retirement centers offer what is called A Life Care Plan or some similar title. This Plan agrees to care for people for the rest of their lives. The purchase of an apartment is usually required, there is a monthly fee charged. These facilities offer all levels of care. When the person's need for care increases they are moved into a part of the facility designed to give the level of care required. The center is under contract to care for a patient even if the patient runs out of money.

Adult Day Care—Many communities now have day care facilities for the elderly. Sometimes these are connected to the Senior Citizens Centers. Sometimes they are facilities built and maintained by the community. The name explains the care. They offer a place for the elderly to be cared for during the day. Most offer great activities and fun. Many are staffed by volunteers who simply love old people and want to help.

Many nursing homes also offer day care. These homes do about the same thing as the community facilities, but since they are not funded by the community nor staffed by volunteers they must charge for these services. The charges are kept to a minimum and the services are usually great.

Respite Care—Some nursing homes will care for your loved one for a week or two at a time to give the caregiver a break. This is a much needed service that far too few caregivers utilize. Some are afraid the parent will be unhappy or resentful. Some are afraid the loved one might get sick while they are gone. Whatever the reasons for not using this idea, it is a great way to find some relief from the constant strain of in-home care. In those cases where it is evident that there is a nursing home stay in the near future, respite care can be a great way to introduce the loved one to the home and give them a chance to get acquainted with the residents and staff. This may make the transition easier.

Assisted Living—My mother was a resident of an assisted living home. She found a peace there that I could only hope for. Assisted living centers do what the name suggests, they help people with living. The staff does not do nursing, but they give the assistance needed to live as normal a life as possible. For example, if a person has trouble dressing themselves the home offers assistance. I know a stock broker who operates his business from an assisted living center. He needs help in some areas of living, but he can use the telephone. With this assistance he continues his career.

Assisted living centers are generally less expensive because they do not offer nursing. Most have a nurse on call or under contract. My mother found living near a nurse stopped her anxiety and fear of getting sick in a house alone.

I recently toured an assisted living center for people with Alzheimer's disease. This lovely facility cared for these patients from the early stages until they needed full nursing home care. Great research went into the design of the building to make the patients feel comfortable and secure.

Nursing Homes—Or Long Term Care Facilities— Different homes use different names but nursing home is the oldest and best known. These facilities have changed dramatically as we have developed better understanding about the needs of the aging. Nursing homes are not warehouses for the aging who are waiting to die. They offer rehabilitation and care that quite often lets a loved one improve enough to return home. Quite often the socialization stimulates a resident to a new way of living. If you have not visited a modern nursing home, you will be amazed at the progress.

Nursing homes now offer different levels of care. Skilled care is one of these levels. Skilled care is rehabilitation. When a person needs to be on a ventilator or is recovering from a surgery or a stroke and needs skilled nursing care, they are placed in the skilled care unit. These units have the ability to do intravenous injections and offer most types of rehabilitative therapies.

What we once called nursing home care now is often called long-term care. Within these facilities there are many variables. Some homes offer upscale sections with more amenities and more privacy. Many have special wings set aside for Alzheimer's patients. These wings are usually staffed with highly trained staff who specialize in the care of people with Alzheimer's disease.

Chapter 12

When Do We Make the Decision?

As soon as I finished speaking a woman's hand shot into the air. She said, "When do you make the decision?" She continued, "I have been shaking for two weeks. I stopped while you were speaking, but I know I will start again. I am an only child and I am responsible for the total care of my mother who has Alzheimer's disease. When do you make the decision?"

I said, "You make the decision when you have been shaking for two weeks." I was trying to convey that there is more involved in the decision than just the condition of the loved one. We also must consider the condition of the caregivers involved. What can they take? What can their health take? What can their families take? What can their marriages take? All of these issues must have as much importance as the condition of the loved one. There is more to the "When" than just whether or not the loved one is bad enough to justify the decision.

Unfortunately most families have a cousin who never married and cared for the parents until they died at ninety-nine and they set the standard by which the whole family is judged. That is comparing apples with oranges. We must have the good sense to evaluate what we are capable of giving and the courage to set those limits in spite of family pressure. It might be in spite of self-imposed pressures.

If we are still struggling with the need for parental approval, we will have a difficult time being honest with ourselves about our limits.

It might be that we wait too long in making these decisions. If a loved one is going to need this kind of help, they usually make a better adjustment if the move is made while they are still able to build a social life. Socialization is one of the best things the home can offer. I have regretted that my mother-in-law did not have the chance to get to know the residents in the home. She loved people and would have been much happier in a social environment.

Parameters

At our family meeting we set some parameters for when my father would become a resident of a care facility. We decided when he could not lift himself so Mother could change his diaper, that would be the time for such a move. When that day came I said, "Let's go tell him." Everyone almost ran out of the house. My own mother would not go into the room with me. I sat by his bed and I told him the truth. I did not tell him we were going for a little ride and let him wake up in a new home. Nor did I tell him it was just for a little while. I told him the truth and I would have done so even if he had been in a coma.

I think our familiy members have the right to honesty.

The fact that the family had talked about and set these parameters was a great deal of help to me when the time came. I knew the family would back up the decision. I knew I was not going to face some members not agreeing and telling my father of their disagreement. The move went smoothly because we had made preparation for it to go smoothly. We faced the "When" question while it was far enough in the future that we could be under less stress and far less emotionally involved. It was easier then and it made it easier when the "When" came.

Chapter 13

End-of-Life Decisions

There is no way to predict what kind of decisions the family might face as the loved one reaches the end of life. Modern medicine has proven to be both a wonderful blessing and a curse. The blessing is we now live longer than any time in history and are on the cusp of curing cancer which will make us live even longer. The curse is that we can live a long time after there is no hope of recovery and no quality of life whatsoever. A physician said, "No one dies of old age anymore. Now we must die of some disease and old age is no longer recognized as a disease." We no longer accept death as a natural end to life. Death is a defeat after a long struggle with some disease. Far too often that struggle is a long fruitless time of great suffering and pain.

I had to decide whether to continue feeding my father. Thankfully, I had given some study to these issues and had talked it over with my father and my family. When the time came, the doctor was honest enough to tell me that our efforts of feeding would only prolong the agony. We stopped the feeding. I had this preparation to lean on and, believe me, I needed it.

We can write living wills and advanced directives and think we have covered every contingency, but when the crunch comes we need to know where the loved one, our families, and even ourselves stand. It is too late for philosophical think sessions. We face a decision that must be made immediately.

Funeral Planning

While the family is together is a good time to begin at least the initial thinking about funeral planning. Families divide over the funeral almost as often as they divide over long-term care decisions. A funeral demands that we make some very tough decisions very quickly while under a great deal of emotional stress. Too often the pressure of time and the emotional stresses can suddenly erupt into a disagreement. The only argument my mother's family ever had was at my grandmother's funeral.

Most of the family members will have ideas about how the funeral should be conducted, who should officiate at the service, and what songs should be sung. Often a family member will have one special thing they especially want done. Many times that member of the family cannot get home as soon as the others and the funeral is planned before they arrive. If the family knows in advance, these special things can be included.

A funeral should be a very personal time of honoring the life of a loved one. Nothing means more to a family than a time of establishing the significance of the person who has died. This can be done much easier and better if the family has had time to think and plan before the need arises. It is hard to think about these things in the hours before the funeral.

We avoid funeral planning because we don't want to think or talk about death or dying. We avoid bringing it up to our aging loved ones because it sounds like we think they are about to die. We are afraid they do not want to talk about it. Most folks want to talk if they only knew how to bring up the subject. Once the ice is broken, they will talk about it with great pleasure.

Since the family is already talking about the future, it is an easy transition to simply suggest that, even though we are a long way from needing such a thing, it would be a good idea to talk about this while we are all together.

The first response from the elderly will usually be, "Oh! Don't go to any trouble or expense." My father said what all fathers say, "Just put me in a box and throw me into a ditch somewhere." I suppose fathers think they are suppose to say that. I said, "Dad, the funeral is our gift to you. I want it to be a gift that shows how much we love you." From that moment on he talked about and planned his funeral with great gusto. He felt like he was loved. He felt like he was in control.

When he died, the family did not have to guess at what he wanted. We sat around and told stories about him and laughed together. The planning was already done.

We were careful to build in some flexibility in the plans. The last thing we want and probably the last thing the loved one would want is a great deal of guilt because we could not follow the plans to the letter. My dad would tell me what he wanted and then with a twinkle in his eye he would say, "Surprise me."

There are some financial considerations involved in funeral planning. If there is going to be a need for Medicaid in the long-term care and the loved one must reduce their worth down to the qualifying level, the government will allow the family to invest in a prepaid funeral plan, and the amount of the investment does not count against the net worth the person must reach to qualify for Medicaid. The amount allowed varies with the different states. Texas, for example, allows $5,000.00. Oklahoma allows $6,000.00. Some states allow prepaid cemetery expenses on top of the allowed figure. The family is not limited to a funeral at that cost. Your funeral director has all of this information and can set up any kind of prearrangement the family may want.

I do not think a family can be over-prepared in these areas. In end of life decisions and funeral planning, the best help available are the decisions the family has already made. The understandings of the past are the basis for making logical decisions even in these emotionally charged settings.

Section Three
The Care Process

Chapter 14

Make Friends With The Physician

If the first step is going to see a lawyer, then the second step is making contact with a physician. Usually a loved one will already be in the care of one or more physicians and there may not be a need to look any further. There may come a time when a specialist will be needed, but that can be arranged through the doctor currently caring for your loved one.

A growing number of physicians specialize in caring for the elderly. They have advanced degrees in geriatric medicine and limit their practice to this area. Since they deal in this area on a full time basis they may have more information than other physicians. They are also willing to care for a patient after a long-term care decision has been made.

From the point when a loved one begins to need some kind of care, every decision about health care must be made in conjunction with a physician. A physician must issue orders for a patient to enter a nursing home and the patient must be under the care of a physician while a resident in the home. Sometimes a person's physician does not work in nursing homes or perhaps doesn't work in the nursing home you have chosen. If so, the nursing home will help you make contact with a physician that has connections with their home. Many nursing homes have a Medical Director who can fulfill these duties.

A physician does not have to issue orders for a person to enter an assisted living center, but the center will require a physical work up and assurance from the physician that the patient is capable of living with this level of care.

It is vitally important that the caregivers build a good relationship with the physician. He or she can be a wonderful help as the hard decisions begin to arrive. Physicians can tell an elderly man that it is time to quit driving his car and get results much faster than one of the children could ever hope for.

The people who attend my conferences do a great deal of complaining about physicians. Not communicating with the family tops the list of these complaints. I guess that is the universal gripe against doctors. Sometimes there are two sides to this issue. Sometimes the physician is just not heard. I have been with families while the doctor did a great job of explaining a procedure and when the doctor left, not a single member of the family had any idea what was said. The family was so intimidated their minds went blank.

Before we go shopping for a new doctor we should be sure the problem is not on our side. Before seeing the physician, write down all of the questions you want answered. Allow the doctor time to speak and then carefully go over each question. Sometimes, if we can calm ourselves down a notch, we may find a great deal of communication coming our way.

There are doctors who will not communicate with the family. If a good effort has been made and communication is not happening, then it is proper and urgent that a change be made.

There are a couple of other issues we need to understand about the medical side of long-term care. First, do not assume the doctor knows about all that is available in long-term care. We hear about too many cases where the doctor said, "Nursing Home" when the patient really needed Assisted Living. The doctor did not know about the availability of such facilities.

Second, if your loved one is showing signs of dementia it is worth the time, effort, and money to have them evaluated. There are many forms of dementia besides Alzheimer's disease. There are also many causes of dementia and some of these cases can be helped.

Chapter 15

No One Wants to Spy On Their Own Parents

We laugh about it in our family. My daughters say they have read my books about long-term care and they now have permission to put us away. So the first time I drool I am going to a home. I know they are joking and I don't feel threatened, but when my wife or I forget something I always say, "Don't tell the kids. They are making a list of those things so they can put us away." All of that is in jest and yet I am finding out the most natural thing in the world for an aging parent to do is to deny they are slipping and to hide the evidence from their children.

Most of the time the family has no idea what condition the parents are in until there is some emergency or some circumstance forces a revelation. The parents may not intend to deceive and may have the children's best interests at heart. They don't want to worry the kids. They don't want the children to have to stop their lives and spend time taking care of them. So they fake how they feel.

Sometimes it is not a fake. When the children come to visit, the parents have a burst of adrenaline and feel much better than normal. Their minds are clear. They have energy. They seem stronger than they were before the children arrived. All of that is a temporary condition that changes as soon as the children leave.

No one wants to spy on their own parents and I certainly am not suggesting such a thing. I do think it is wise for the family to find ways of monitoring the condition of aging loved ones. Monitoring is more a process of learning to watch and to listen. It is not prying nor breaking into the private world of a loved one. We just need to look and listen.

The kitchen can tell us a great deal. Burned pans can mean our loved one is forgetting that the stove is on. The condition of the food in the refrigerator is another very subtle clue to the changing conditions in the home.

The overall look of the home is important. As we age we are not able to keep our homes in the same condition as we could when we were young. Allowances must be made for aging, but the overall look can give some great clues. Burn marks on the furniture, or dirty dishes left in unusual places can signal the onset of dementia.

The physical appearance is also a great clue. Notice if they are bathing properly or getting very careless about clothing or not grooming in their usual way and seem to not care how they look. Watch for bruises that could indicate far too many unreported falls in the home.

If your parents are convinced they have won the

sweepstakes it is a good idea to notice if there are far too many magazines laying around. The elderly are easily deluded by the promises with print so small they cannot possibly read it. Too many magazines are not only costly, but they may indicate your loved one is an easy prey to the scam artists who prey on the elderly. The magazines can mean it is time to take a hard look at your loved one's ability to handle money. This may mean it is time for someone to start helping with the checkbook while taking great care to let them do everything they can for themselves. We can be the second opinion they can turn to when faced with hard decisions.

I am sixty-six years old. I have stopped doing business over the phone. Telemarketers are wasting their time and I tell them if they want to sell me something they should send it through the mail. I have taken this hard stand in the hope that as I grow older I will maintain that stance and not be available to the scam artist. In the future I plan to set up my accounts so a check for an amount over $200.00 must be co-signed by one of my children. That sounds drastic, but in my world I hear far too many accounts of folks losing their life savings because their ability to discern has diminished and the family never noticed.

A casual visit with the neighbors can tell you more about what is really going on with your parents than almost anything I know. Neighbors know if they are able to get out or are isolating themselves inside the house.

Neighbors know how well they can drive. They know if they have fallen in the yard. They know if they are forgetting where they live. They know if their personalities are changing in drastic ways.

If the loved ones have always bought groceries at the same store, a talk with the grocer can also be revealing.

I think a private visit with your loved one's physician is a good idea. Not only can they help you understand what is happening to your loved one, but you can give information to the doctor that will not be discovered in any other way. Too often we take our loved ones to the doctor and there is no time or method for us to tell him what is happening at home. We don't want to say too much in front of our loved one, so we just hope the doctor can read our minds—they can't.

As I say, being a spy on our loved ones does not feel very good, but as they get older we need more information than they will tell us and their condition can get out of hand before we know what's happening.

Chapter 16

If Care Is Needed

When it becomes evident there will be a time when a loved one can no longer stay at home, then it is time to start searching for a long-term solution to their care. These logical steps to follow will help in seeking the proper solution. The first step is to review the section of this book on the levels of care. Now is the time to match the needs of your loved one with the types of care available. The choices can range from getting help in the loved one's home, moving them to one of the children's homes, or moving to some type of long-term care facility. The choice becomes easier if you know the types of services that are available in your community.

Where to Find Help

Most families do not know where to even begin searching for the available facilities. Fortunately in most cities or counties there is a great deal of free help just waiting for a call. The Area Agency On Aging program covers almost all of the United States. There are similar programs in Canada. These agencies offer a complete list of all of the care facilities as well as other pertinent services such as attorneys, physicians, day care and home health care. More detailed information about these agencies can be found in the Tool Chest section of this book.

Many communities will have people who are now making themselves available to walk with families through these decisions and serve the family as needed after the decision is made. These people go under a variety of titles from Elder Care Case Manager to Placement Consultants. Most nursing homes know about these people and will refer families to them. The Area Agency On Aging will also know of the availability of this type of service.

These consultants can be invaluable. They have intimate knowledge of every facility in the city and can help match the facility to the family. They also offer a great service to families who live in another city and need someone to check on the condition and care of the loved one. They can give the family a great sense of relief and insure proper care of the loved one. Some of these companies offer such added services as transportation to doctor visits, in-home visits and service, and bonded bookkeeping for elderly loved ones.

If your loved one is showing signs of dementia, a visit with the nearest Alzheimer's Association is worthwhile. I am amazed at how many families tell me they think their loved one might have Alzheimer's, but when I question them I find they have not been to a doctor for an evaluation or to the Alzheimer's Association for information. Alzheimer's seems to generate a fear of facing reality and a sense that if we never hear the actual diagnosis then maybe it won't be so. As I have already mentioned, dementia comes in many forms and has many causes. Some types of dementia can be treated with a great deal of success. I know of no better place to find information and support than the Alzheimer's Associations around the country. To find the nearest chapter call 1-800-272-3900. There is even a web sight: www.alz.org.

Chapter 17

How to Select a Care Facility

There is no great secret in selecting a facility to care for an aging loved one, and there are some great resources available to help in the quest. As reported in the last chapter, a call to the Area Agency On Aging is a great place to start. The Ombudsman program will provide a list of care facilities along with a report of the regular inspections all nursing homes are given. This is a good method of finding the location of the available care in a given area.

I would give a word of caution about the rating report. When a nursing home is inspected they may receive a number of deficiencies. On the surface it would seem that a number of deficiencies would automatically indicate a bad nursing home. The problem is the inspectors only have one word to use for all kinds of problems. A deficiency can be anything from giving the wrong medication to putting a soft drink in the refrigerator and not recording when it was placed there. Needless to say the wrong medication is very serious but the soft drink might not be quite as life threatening. Both are called a deficiency. A large number of deficiencies is a red flag but not an automatic disqualification.

I was glad to see the development of family consultants begin to happen. These folks can help families with the tough decisions and serve as a bridge between the facility and the family. These are especially helpful when the family does not live in the same city as the parents. Most of the time parents want to stay in the city where they live and these consultants can make that work very well.

Even with all of the help available it still comes down to the family members getting the feel of the place. "Feel of the place" is a good choice of terms. That is exactly what we should look for. We should not go into the home like a mother-in-law searching for dust. We should go there with our feelers out. Try to catch the spirit of the place. I can walk through a nursing home and almost immediately know whether I want one of my loved ones living there. I look for staff that seem happy and have a sense of humor. I notice whether they touch the residents. I have walked through nursing homes with administrators who hugged every resident they saw and it was evident this was not their first time to hug. The residents lit up when they approached and were in hugging position when they got there. That is what I am looking for.

As aging began to appear my mother would say, "If I have to go will you be sure it is a nice one?" She wanted a place she could be proud of. The building matters. The design of a building can add much to the comfort and safety of a loved one.

The location matters. It helps if the family can be close enough for regular visits. It is also important that the lifelong friends have access also.

Notice the smell, but give it a second chance. Every nursing home smells occasionally. Incontinent people live there. If the smell is there on the second visit then I think it is a definite mark against that home.

I think every family should visit the nursing home at least twice. The first visit should be arranged in advance. The second time they should just drop in at lunch time and, if possible, eat in the dining room. The loudest complaint your loved one will voice will be about the food. The strange thing is most folks living in a nursing home are much better fed than they were while living at home alone. Finding the motivation to cook is hard for folks who live alone. Sometimes it is hard for elderly couples to find the energy to prepare proper meals.

Finances must be considered in making the choice. If your loved one will need the help of Medicaid then the family must find a nursing home that accepts this form of payment. Some nursing homes are not certified to accept Medicaid patients. In many cases the family will start out the care as private pay with the realization that the money will run out. When this happens the loved one will need to become a Medicaid patient. If that is a possibility then a home should be selected that qualifies for Medicaid.

Then, when the time comes, the loved one will not have to move to another facility and be forced to leave their social life for a second time.

A nursing home must have orders from a physician before they can admit a resident. The resident must have a physician who will agree to take them as a patient while they are in the nursing home. More and more nursing homes have contracts with staff physicians who are available to the residents of that home. This is a great asset to the resident and to the family. Most of the time the resident can have a doctor's care right in the nursing home without the need of an office visit. The availability of medical care is also one of the vital issues in choosing a facility.

A check list of things to look for in making the nursing home choice is included in the Tool Chest section of this book.

Chapter 18

Planning the Move

Planning the move requires careful thought. Even moving into the home of a family member, should be carefully planned. What should be taken and what must be left become traumatic choices for the loved one. Many loved items must stay behind. A great deal of the grief the loved one will feel comes from the loss of well-loved possessions that must be left behind. There will be things that could not be given away at a rummage sale that are priceless treasures to the loved one.

We were fortunate in the cases of both my mother-in-law and my mother. We were not forced to sell either of their houses when the move happened. They were able to participate in the distribution of their possessions. My mother-in-law said she wanted to live long enough to get even with her children. She got even by enjoying our struggle in deciding what to do with a lifelong collection of things. We would make a weekend trip to work on her house. On our return she would listen to each detail and each struggle with great interest and joy.

In both cases the making of decisions about who got each item gave our loved ones something to engage their minds and something to enjoy. It also gave them a sense of being a vital part in the decisions about what happened to them as well as to their stuff.

Adjusting to Life in a Care Facility

A person who becomes a resident of a care facility will go through a period of adjustment. They will go through some grieving and they should be allowed to do so. Quite often I think the loved ones get through the adjustment better than the family. Sometimes we feel so guilty we cannot see how well they're doing. Sometimes they learn how to manipulate us by not doing well when we are there and doing wonderfully when we're absent. It pays to consult with the staff about how well the adjustment is going. I have heard far too many stories of mothers who are just withering away crying in their rooms only to find when the family is not around the mother is the social secretary for the whole facility.

During the first week of stay the family needs to visit but not stay long. That is one of those "tough love" sort of things. The loved one needs to begin forming a social life and is much more likely to do so if the family is not furnishing it for them. The danger is that the family will become the social life and will be expected to maintain a constant presence for the rest of the stay.

It is also important that we not begin doing too much for our loved one. Whatever job you start will become your job forever. Your loved one will want you to do it instead of the staff. The staff will get in the habit of your doing it and not remember to check to see if it has been done. Your loved one will get much better care if it is clear from the very beginning that the needed services will be done by the staff and not be taken over by the family. The first week is the best time to establish how the care will be given and who is responsible.

Roles

Most families do not establish what will be done by the staff in the facility and what will be done by the family. A good easy answer is to let the staff take care of the physical needs and the family be the connection with the outside world. The family can help keep the loved one living in the present and keep their minds alert and active. Visits should not be a time for taking over the job you are paying the facility to provide. They should not be times when all of the time is spent checking for mistakes or slights. Visits should be times for the family to bring in news from the outside world to share with a loved one.

While I was an active minister I spoke for a retirement center once each month. I rarely missed my turn because I enjoyed the folks so much. I liked them even more because they seemed to enjoy my visits and often would tell me how my talks were the best of all. I thought that was mostly flattery and that they probably said that to all of the speakers. Then the chaplain told me they were saying the same thing to him when I was not around. I finally asked them what they found enjoyable about my talks. They said I was the only one who seemed to think they were still interested in what was happening in the world. They said most of the other speakers talked only about death and heaven, while I talked about current events and even discussed hard theological ideas with them. Often I would tell them where I was going to speak and what I was going to talk about. When I returned I would tell them about the trip. Sometimes we discussed geography so long that there was no time for my speech. I had accidentally found a key. I connected them with the outside world and it had meaning to them.

A family can do the same. Take family pictures. Make a running list of family events in between visits. Even the most trivial will have meaning. Talking about an upcoming trip will not make them sad because they cannot go, it will make them feel involved and an important part of the family.

I know a woman who took the various materials and pictures to her mother's room and together they built a family calendar. Each family birthday featured a picture of the person who was being honored. The calendar had large spaces for each day so the family members could sign on the day of their visits. This does wonders when the loved one tends to complain about no one coming to visit them. Each time the woman came to visit she would bring mementos of family events to put on the calendar. This is but one of thousands of creative ideas that can help keep the loved one attached to the outside world and make visits an adventure instead of a chore.

The family can be the source of a positive attitude about the facility. If family members feel overwhelmed with guilt they tend to notice every negative thing about the care and the facility. That attitude rubs off on the loved one. If the family is positive and spend their time enjoying the loved one and keeping the communication alive, the loved one will be more positive also.

Chapter 19

Building Communication

"Why won't they listen to me? I've told them and told them and they just don't hear. It is evident they can no longer take care of themselves, but when I say anything they just get mad." "When did I become the bad guy? I have always been a good daughter and all of a sudden I am the enemy. What have I done to deserve that?"

I hear those statements and worse at almost every conference. Something happens to communication and we are left with anger, hurt, and guilt. Learning to communicate with our elderly loved ones may be the most important issue we can face. The kind of care they receive is vital, of course, but if communication breaks down the greatest care in the world will not bring peace to either our loved one or ourselves.

Communication must begin by our walking a mile in their shoes. We must understand what they are experiencing and feeling. There are several changes going on that they cannot explain even to themselves, but have an effect on how they relate to us.

They are Afraid of Losing Control

Growing old is a gradual loss of control. It feels as if they are no longer the captain of their ship. It feels as though they have to ask permission before they can do anything. They can't just go on a trip anymore. Now they must consult the doctor, arrange for medications, and be sure the accommodations are all right. Then they realize they can't drive as long or as well as they once did. The children are upset because they are going alone. Suddenly they have to ask the children if it is all right to go on a trip. They are slowly losing control of their lives and it is scary. How much control will they lose? How helpless will they become? What kind of life will others allow?

When the roles change and we become parent to our parents we lose the ability to communicate and must build it back again in a new relationship. This phenomenon can be seen in any nursing home. A family can't stay in the room with their loved one more than two minutes, but they can go next door and visit with a total stranger all afternoon. Some families find it so uncomfortable that it becomes difficult to visit. Some won't go at all.

This loss of communication is a natural thing. Anytime we experience role changes we must learn to communicate in the new roles. I discovered what impact this loss of communication can have when I became parent to my father. Suddenly, I found it difficult and uncomfortable being around him. We went from being wonderfully close friends to total strangers. When he came for a visit, I hoped he would not stay long, and I had to force myself to go see him. The guilt of these feelings became almost overwhelming to me. I wondered what happened, and if I no longer loved my father. I finally confronted my father with these feelings and found out he didn't like me either. He felt that I was taking over his life. It felt to him like it would feel to a forty-five year-old woman whose mother had just told her how to keep house. He resented the loss of control.

A woman said, "That explains why my father, who has always been the kindest man I ever knew, is now being mean to me. He is fighting me. He does not want me to be his parent."

This also can be a cause of guilt. The communication dies between the parent and the child who becomes the parent, but it doesn't necessarily do so between the rest of the family. Suddenly this one child is the object of anger and even abuse while the rest of the family looks on in disbelief. In dysfunctional families some siblings might respond with glee.

The loved one is losing control and the ones who seem to be gaining control become the objects of anger and rejection. This has a profound effect on how we communicate.

There is Grief in Aging

Grief doesn't just happen when someone dies. Grief is the natural response to any loss. There is loss in aging. Matter of fact that is what aging is—the slow process of losing who we are. One of the natural responses to grief is anger. Grief causes feelings of frustration, fear, rejection, hurt, and disappointment. These are all forms of anger. Anger needs to be expressed, but it is difficult to find anyone who will listen and understand. Too often instead of expressing anger, they tend to just stop communicating. We are left wondering what happened.

While this chapter has been aimed primarily at the communication between the parents and their children, the same loss of communication happens between husbands and wives. The husband suddenly goes from being the strong provider to having to be cared for by his wife. Quite often the anger and grief he feels can focus on his wife. When this happens, long standing communication patterns are changed and too often we don't know how to establish any new ones. Harsh words can replace the loving responses the couple once knew.

Communicating with our elderly loved ones must begin with our understanding that some very traumatic things are happening in their lives. These events will have an effect on how they relate and communicate with us. If we do not understand these changes it is easy to allow the guilt and frustration to cut off any hope of communication.

Walk in Your Shoes

There are also some things going on inside of us that affect our ability to communicate with our parents. It is hard to talk with your parents when you know they do not want to hear what you are going to say. It is hard to be around them when you feel like they disapprove of you or are angry with you.

No matter how long we have been away from home.
No matter how strong a person we have become.
No matter how independent we are.

When a parent starts expressing disapproval, disappointment, or disagreement we become little children seeking approval. That is the normal reaction we have to our parents.

Parent/Child

Sometimes our relationship with our parents intensifies this normal reaction. Some of us have never built an adult-to-adult relationship with our parents. We are still their little boy or girl. The hardest thing about being a parent is learning how to quit being one. When I said that at a conference a lady said, "My mother is past eighty and was seriously injured in a car wreck. When I went into the emergency room to see her, she opened one eye and said, 'When are you going to do something about that hair?'" Now that is mothering to the bitter end. Unfortunately most relationships remain parent to child. We need to build an adult to adult relationship with our parents even if we must do so by force of will. If not, they will continue to parent and we will continue to resist and feel guilty because we resisted. If a parent continues to be the parent after the child is grown, the only tools they have to use in the effort are guilt producing. They can pout, they can hint, or they can whine. Any of these three leave them miserable because they don't work, and they leave us miserable for the same reason.

Culture

A man I met on an airplane got defensive when he learned what kind of books I wrote. He said he was Greek and that his culture demanded that the eldest son take care of the parents until they died. He was the eldest son and his father had moved into his home. He said, "He will have a home in my home until he dies." I said, "I appreciate your culture, but your father may outlive your ability to do that. He may need more care than you can give. If he develops Alzheimer's he will outlive your ability to do that. With Alzheimer's it is not whether you will make a nursing home decision it is when you will do so." He touched my arm and said, "It is already happening. And to make matters worse, I am in a second marriage and have a new son. How do you find a nanny that will care for an old man and a baby at the same time?"

When our culture is screaming at us and we feel trapped, we find it hard to communicate or relate. Our own guilt colors our every view and thought. Talking to our parents about breaking those cultural norms is more than difficult, it is frightening.

How Am I Suppose to Feel?

Some will have a great struggle with guilt because they do not know how they are suppose to feel. I wrote a small book called <u>Searching For Normal Feelings</u> which tries to show how deeply we struggle trying to find out what is normal for us to feel. We seem to think we are suppose to feel a certain way about our parents no matter what our relationship with them happens to be. We especially feel this when they become old or ill.

I met a man in New Zealand who said, "How could I feel like my father is a burden? What kind of son am I to think that about a father who gave his life to support my family?" When we are called on to give full time care to our parents they are a burden, and it is normal to feel that they are.

We need to understand that we love them but we still get angry and tired and frustrated. Having those feelings does not mean we don't love them. It simply means we are in a tiring and frustrating situation that leaves us with mixed feelings. If you are a parent then you can remember the first months of a child's life when you spent all of your time feeding, washing, cleaning, and comforting the newborn child. You loved them with all of your being, and yet you were often tired, frustrated and numb. It is normal to feel burdened when you are burdened.

When we don't feel the way we think we are supposed to feel, we begin to think there is something wrong with us. This can lead us to become over-compensators who try to hide how we feel by over-doing the care of a loved one.

A physician asked me to see a woman who was about to have a nervous breakdown caring for her mother who was a resident of a nursing home. Her mother had been in the home for more than seven years. The woman took meals to her mother every day. She washed the sheets on the beds even though they had just been washed. She complained to the staff constantly about the care of her mother. She seemed to be the most protective and caring person possible. She had almost wrecked her marriage in the process. Her health was deteriorating and her children would not come to see her because they did not want to hear about how badly they were neglecting their grandmother.

The first time we visited I said, "I want you to tell me how you really feel about your mother. I promise I will never tell anyone else but I want you to tell me." She could not do it. She came seven times before she could tell me and then she said, "I am going to tell you and then lightening is going to strike me dead." Then she said, "My mother has been an alcoholic most of my life and I wish I never had to see her again." She cannot deal with those feelings so she hides them behind a facade of over-doing and over-caring to the point of exhaustion.

Unfinished Agendas

Some of us come to this time of life with a lot of old scars and pains that we have never been able to confront or get past. These can make us feel a great deal of guilt or drive us away from caring. It would be wonderful if we could have a great time of confrontation and healing between our parents and ourselves and finish those old agendas. That may happen in some cases, but in most cases this ideal cannot be reached. The substitute for this time of healing is for the family to hear and understand our feelings. Grudges don't happen because someone is too hard-headed to forgive. Grudges happen when our hurts are ignored or trivialized and they become obsessions to us. This is a great time for brothers and sisters to lay aside the old baggage of the past and hear one another's stories. There is healing in the hearing.

Not everyone who reads this will fit one of the types of relationships mentioned here. Some will have had a warm and accepting family and these struggles will seem quite foreign. No matter what kind of relationship you may have had in the past, there will now be the need for a new kind of communication. The issues we must face now will force us to communicate under a great deal of stress.

Chapter 20

The Unblessed Child

Some folks are dealing with a lifelong feeling of being the unblessed child. It seems as though almost every family will have one child that just does not feel blessed. They don't think they are as attractive or intelligent or talented as the other children in the home. Many times children raised as an only child feel like they have never lived up to their parent's expectations for them. Some unblessed children leave home and try to forget the past. Most never leave. They stay home and spend the rest of their lives trying to earn the blessing. I know fifty-year-old women who go see their mothers every day and every day their mothers tell them how great the other children are. Never how great they are.

A woman told me how excited she was to have found the perfect Christmas gift for her mother. She said her mother had never acknowledged any gift she had bought for her in the past but this time it would be different. The gift was so expensive she had put it in lay-a-way and was going to spend six months paying it off. She said it was a good thing the gift was not available because if it were she could not wait until Christmas to give it to her mother. When Christmas arrived, she presented her gift and her mother **never said a word**. The woman has a sister who lives in another state and has very little contact with her mother. The sister sent a handkerchief which the mother put in a frame and hung on the wall. The mother points out the handkerchief to every person who comes by and never says a word about the gift from the unblessed local daughter who is desperate for some kind of notice and blessing.

It is amazing how often the unblessed child becomes the primary caregiver to the elderly parents. It happens because they still live near the home or will return. If an unblessed child must leave home physically, they never leave emotionally. The first sign of illness and they are back. It also happens because the unblessed child sees this as their chance to serve and be recognized and loved. Unfortunately it doesn't happen that way.

Sometimes the sense of inferiority and lack of worth comes from siblings. A woman said, "I have to work. My sister lives here in town and does not work. I have total care of our mother. Sister does not help, not even financially. I work for an accountant and, because of changes in the tax laws, we got behind in our work and I had to ask for some help. My sister agreed to take Mother for two weeks so I could get caught up on work. After one week she called and said, 'Come and get this woman, she is driving me insane.' When I went after Mother, my sister met me on the front porch and said, 'Don't you dare put my mother in a nursing home.'"

I said to that lady what I say to unblessed children all over the country. "Why do you let people treat you like that? No one can put that kind of guilt on you without your permission. Manipulation is by invitation only. The only answer for the unblessed child is to stand up and say, 'This is me. Decide right now whether or not you want to love me. If you do, fine. If not, I will learn to live without it, but I am not going to spend another day chasing a rainbow that has no pot of gold at the end of it.'"

Chapter 21

Gifts That Communicate

Hopefully we have walked in enough shoes to understand what we are experiencing and what must be overcome before communication can be established. Now the question is how do we bridge these gaps or, in some cases, chasms and find mutual ground upon which we can build new relationships? May I suggest a couple of gifts that can do wonders in building the miracle of communication.

The Gift of Significance

If I could give any gifts to my loved ones I would begin with the gift of significance. When things happen to us the first thing we want and need to do is establish the significance of that event. If someone witnesses a horrible accident, the first thing they will tell is how scared they were and what it did to them. That is not selfishness, it is human nature. If a child has a hurt hand, they will want a bandage on it no matter whether it is needed or not. Then they will show everyone their hurt. After everyone has seen the hurt and made an appropriate response the bandage can be removed and the incident forgotten. If someone refuses to stop and look at the hurt, the child will kick them in the shins. The hurt must be seen. That is how we deal with hurts. It cannot be forgotten until the significance of the hurt has been acknowledged.

Imagine your mother's house. She has lived there for many years. She has treasures there that you could not give away at a rummage sale. Suddenly she is old. Or her health is failing. She must move from her home. Where she moves doesn't matter, the needs and the feelings are the same. She is going to lose some things. She will lose most of her stuff. She will lose her social life. She will lose the traditions of her life. Those things she always did at Christmas, Easter, Hanukkah, or other meaningful days in her life.

She wants to establish the significance of those losses. When she tries, our natural tendency is to change the subject. We want her to be positive. We don't want to hear any tears or complaints, so we begin to tell her how much better things are going to be. She realizes we will not let her establish the significance so she tries to tell others. They don't want to talk about it either. Gradually the loss becomes an obsession she cannot move past.

Significance is another way of saying understanding. We just want our thoughts and feelings understood. To have someone give credence to our thoughts and legitimize our feelings is healthy. We don't need any explanations or cheering up. We just want to be heard and understood. The opposite of understanding is not misunderstanding—it is trivialization. We trivialize when we put the best face on the situation. We trivialize when we avoid talking about it.

At a recent conference a man said, "My father had to

leave the farm where not only he was born, but his father was also born there. The farm had deep significance in his life, but there was no other choice. He keeps wanting to talk about it and I have been afraid it would make him feel worse so I always change the subject. You are saying it would be better and more healing if I let him talk about the farm."

How else can he establish the significance of his loss unless someone understands his feelings about that loss and lets him talk it out?

Two sisters came to a conference terribly upset. They talked with great anger about their mother who would not listen to them and would not do what it was evident she needed to do. When I talked about significance one almost shouted at me. "I have done that. I told her I knew she had feelings. I have feelings too. I told her she would feel the same no matter where she lived." At the next "I told her" I interrupted to say, "There is a difference in telling and understanding, and you can't do both. You must decide whether you are going to spend the rest of your mother's days in explanations or in communication. Communication starts when we are willing to understand and give significance to their pain."

While we have been talking about children and parents, the same principles work between mates. We get so busy telling our mates how they should feel or think that we never try to understand and never give the gift of significance.

By the way, the members of the family are also suffering losses and pain. Nothing can bring more healing than family members sharing with one another and giving the gift of significance. Remember, we cannot change the way people feel by changing the way they think. Hear and understand.

The Gift of Anger

I would also give the gift of anger. My mother had to go to the nursing home with a broken pelvis. She was only going to be there for eight weeks. She knew about the length of her stay and knew the doctor had made the decision that she become a resident of the home. Every time I went to see her she would say things to make me feel guilty. She did not want to attack me so she would complain about the nursing home and make me feel bad because she was there. I know better, but I would react every time, and respond with some idea prefaced by "Now Mother you know..." We should get that phrase out of our vocabularies. There is nothing we can say that is good after we have said it. It means "I am getting ready to trivialize you."

I would say, "You know you are only here for eight weeks. You know the doctor made you come. You know this is the best nursing home in town." One day I woke up to what I was doing. When she started the guilt trip I pulled my chair up close and said, "You are angry about being in here, aren't you?"

She said "Yes, and I should be bigger than that. Every day when you leave I swear I am not going to do that anymore, but when you walk in it just seems to come out."

I said, "Mom it is all right to be angry. If I have to come here to live I am going to be angry. And it is all right to tell me you are angry." From that day until the day she died, I gave her the gift of anger. What a gift.

Chapter 22

Taking Care of You

A professor in a school of mines asked his class to decide what was the most important thing to ever come out of the mines. They guessed gold, diamonds, platinum and other valuable minerals. The professor said, "The most important thing to come out of the mines is the miner." We have talked a great deal about decision making and long-term care issues, but the real challenge in long-term care is caring for those who must give the care.

Far too often the caregiver dies before the patient. Everyone knows of cases when a mate was in very poor health and the spouse succumbed to the stress and work of the caring. I see spouses at the seminars that are under so much stress I wonder how much longer they can last.

I see too many cases where the caregiver hangs on beyond what is good for the loved one. This is more prevalent among spouses, but family members also go too far.

I can't relate how many times someone has asked, "How do you know when you have had all you can take?" Earlier in this book we listed a bill of rights for the family to follow in supporting the primary caregiver. Now we need a bill of rights for us to use on ourselves.

1. **Why are you doing the work in the first place?** If you are doing it in some effort to become loved by your family, then you are in danger of being one who over-does and over-compensates. This is not the time for curing unblessed child syndrome. This is a time of giving care because you chose to do so in order to meet a need in the family.

2. **Don't do it because you were pressured by the family.** Some folks have never learned how to stand up to their family and are easily talked or bullied into care. Just because you are the only girl in the family does not automatically volunteer you to be the caregiver. Your reasons for serving or not serving are just as valid and important as anyone else's.

3. **Don't be driven by culture.** This is especially true of husbands taking care of wives. We men have always been the ones who fix things and take care of the family. This can become something you can't fix. There might come a time when they need more care than you can give. That does not make you a failure. That does not mean you did not live up to your vows to care through sickness and health till death do you part. Sometimes caring means letting those who can give the best care take over.

4. **When offered a break—take it.** Sometimes a family offers help and the primary caregiver will not accept their offer. It is easy to become indispensable. It is easy to decide the loved one could not live if you were not there. Take a break.

5. Watch your feelings. There is a form of depression that does not exemplify itself by blue feelings. This depression leaves you with no feelings. You feel detached. You feel as if you are standing outside of yourself and watching as you go through the motions. You can't seem to drum up any emotional response to anything. All of us have days when we feel detached and nonresponsive, but if the condition persists it means you are depressed and you need a break. This is the time for giving yourself some tender loving care. This is a warning flag that tells you to stop being wonderful and noble and go take a rest.

6. Let others help you cope. There is such a thing as the care-givers syndrome. We get very good at giving care and never learn to receive it. Every caregiver has some caregiver syndrome in them. Some of us have a whole lot of it. I have a bad case myself. I am working on it and am better, but I can sit up with someone and listen to their pain all night. I can listen. I can understand. I can give them significance. But if I sat up all night they would never know of my pain. I wouldn't tell them. The syndrome folks hide their own pain while they work on everyone else's.

The hardest part of loving to those of us so afflicted is not in loving, it is in being loved. I think it is a form of being in control. Someone can ask about some problem in my life and I will immediately say, "Tell me, how are you doing?" I don't want to be vulnerable. I have to to be the healer. I can't be the heal-ee. I have to bless people. I can't let them bless me.

We love to hear "You are doing too much." That is like saying "sic'em" to a bull dog. We will work that much harder hoping they will say it again. We get our jollies out of being the ones who serve.

The healthiest day of my life was the day after my brother died when I decided to cut a trip short, miss an important meeting, and fly home so someone else could take care of me. We are only healthy when we know how to let someone else take care of us. It is not enough to know how to love. It is only enough when you know how to be loved in return.

The Tool Chest

After writing this material I thought it would be a good idea to try to make this book as practical and easy to use as possible. When we are deeply involved in this process we don't have time for philosophical ideas. We need to know how to get the job done. I live in Oklahoma City which would be considered to be a medium-sized city. I set out to find all of the resources I could find here to help me make these decisions. I am including many of the ones I thought to be the most helpful.

I immediately discovered one of the greatest resources of all. I called the office of The Area Agency On Aging. There is either an office or a phone number to cover every county in our state and I understand this is true all over the United States. I received a 200 page book called <u>Survival Kit For Seniors</u>. I understand each agency has something like this book. It lists every known group, person, government agency, support group, and place to file complaints in the county and state. I was amazed to find they also have an Ombudsman program to help insure good care from nursing facilities. There is no need for any family to face this decision alone. Help is a phone call away. I even found a national 800 number for The Elder Care Locator which will furnish information about senior services in every area of the United States. The number is 1-800-677-1116. I am sure there are helps of this type available throughout Canada.

I interviewed some of these resource people and got permission to publish some of the tools they use in helping people. I am not including interviews with the professions we automatically know about and know how to find. I am not including interviews with lawyers, physicians, or long-term care professionals. These are obvious and available. I chose the helps we might not know about or know how to find. I am including the ones that could most likely be found in most cities or counties.

The people I called for interviews are actively involved in selling their products or services and I list their companies. This does not in any way suggest that you should purchase these services from these companies and should not be considered an endorsement from me. I just stumbled on to these folks. I am sure there are many others just as qualified and whose products are just as good. I asked each one to tell me about the product or service and to make every effort not to slant the interview toward their particular brand or company. I think the ones included here did a good job of being bipartisan and fair.

Each one expressed the hope that their contribution would be of service to those who use this book in the process of care.

SANDRA'S LISTS

One of the first and most helpful of the interviews was with a Geriatric Case Manager named Sandra Sherry. Sandra has started a company to help families in long-term care. She walks the family through the decision making process and, if a care facility is needed, she has information on each one. She tries to guide a family to the facility that fits them best. She knows the ins-and-outs of Medicaid and insurance. She knows what the facilities charge and which ones take Medicaid.

One of her most important services is to those families who live a distance from their aging parents. She will visit the parents on a regular basis, transport them to doctors appointments and do other such needed services. She keeps the family posted on the condition of the loved ones and, if a care facility is needed, she will help them with the placement and then continue to monitor both the loved one and the facility. This is a new and growing field. It will not be long before these folks will be available everywhere. They may go by different titles but they all offer much the same services.

Sandra was kind enough to allow me to use five of her check lists. I hope you find them helpful.

CHECKLIST FOR MOVING A LOVED ONE INTO YOUR HOME

1. Do you have a full time job?
2. Is there someone at home to be with the family member during the day?
3. Does your house have wide enough doors for wheel chair access?
4. Is your bathtub elderly accessible?
5. Is your car easily accessible for the elderly?
6. If not, are funds available to make the house and car accessible?
7. Will a child be moved out of his/her room to make room for the family member?
8. What is the family schedule? Are you busy most evenings? Do the children take up most of your time?
9. If you are single, what is your life style? Do you enjoy being able to set your own schedule and not answer to anyone?
10. How strong is your marriage?
11. What is your relationship with your elderly loved one?

These are simple questions. They are not presented to make a family think they should not move a loved one into their home. They are asked so a family can think through the issues before making such a move. Too often the move is made and then the thinking is done. Too many families operate on "ready—fire—aim."

The most important question is number 11. If the relationship has not been good, then it may be questionable whether to make this choice. The relationship is not going to suddenly improve. Matter of fact, it might get worse. The loved one may resent being out of control. You may find them infuriating at times. The life-style of the family must change and that can cause resentment. These issues need to be faced with honesty and courage before the decision is made.

If the decision to move the loved one into your home is not the right one to make, it takes courage, but I hope you will find enough to do what is best instead of what is easiest. Love is doing what people need, not what they want.

CHECKLIST FOR INITIAL VISIT TO A CARE FACILITY

We should not go into the facility like a mother-in-law looking for dust, but we should have some kind of checklist to help us compare the sites on an initial impression basis. We are really looking for the spirit of the place. Some items on the list might not be just right on the day of the visit, but if the spirit is right then go back for a second look.

1. Is the general atmosphere warm and happy?
2. Is the staff courteous helpful and caring toward the residents?
3. Is there a clean smell as you walk in the door?
4. If no, does it smell like urine?
5. Do residents seem content and well groomed?
6. Is the office staff friendly and helpful in showing the facility?
7. Are the outside grounds well kept?
8. Is there a place for families to visit outside of the rooms?
9. Is there a copy of the residents rights posted in each room?
10. Are the call buttons convenient and easy to reach?
11. Is the facility licensed to accept Medicaid?
12. Are activities planned for each day of the week including weekends?
13. Are there activities for the inactive and bedridden residents?
14. Are religious services offered?

15. Does the facility meet the standards for number of staff on each floor?
16. Is the dining room attractive and inviting?
17. Are special dietary needs met?
18. How many beds are in the facility?
19. Is there a waiting list?
20. Does the home accept Alzheimer's residents?
21. Does the home encourage family participation?

SELECTING A CARE FACILITY

If your loved one is in need of a nursing home there are some things to consider and some things you need to know. This is the time for looking deeper than the first check list and discovering the information that directly effects the care.

Things to Consider

Location Which area of the city will be best and most convenient? In cases of families in small towns there may, of necessity, be a decision between having a loved one close by or choosing a larger and more comprehensive facility in another city. The family being close by is of value and each family must weigh this against the type of care available.

Size and Cost If there are several facilities to choose from, make a list of four or five to be considered. Call each to find out about the size, (they use the number of beds), the cost per room, if the site accepts Medicaid, and if rooms are available. If the family member has been diagnosed with Alzheimer's or if you suspect that will be the diagnosis, find out if the home accepts Alzheimer's residents.

What the homes are like Narrow your choice to two or three facilities. Visit each at least twice. One visit by schedule, the other without their knowing you are coming. If possible, take your loved one with you. If they feel like they are part of the decision they will much more readily accept the transition.

Things You Need to Know

- **Staff/ resident ratio** Your Area Agency On Aging can furnish the regulations for your state. See if the site meets these regulations.

- **Activities** What type of activities are provided? Are they available on evenings and weekends? Are they available to the residents who cannot get out of bed?

- **Direct Care Staff** Are the nursing assistants certified according to state requirements?

- **Number of Beds** The size of the facility does not determine the quality of the care, but it is wise to match the site with the comfort level of the family member. If they have trouble with large crowds, then maybe a smaller home should be considered.

- **Medicaid Certified** If your loved one will need this help at any time in the future, it is best to chose a home that is so certified. Otherwise you will face a move when the need arises.

- **Staff doctor** Every facility must have a staff physician to oversee the medical care in the home. You need to find out if your family member's doctor will go to the facility you have chosen. Everyone who becomes a resident of a nursing home must enter on doctor's orders and must be under a doctor's care while in the facility.

- **Ratio of Nurses on the Floor** Every state requires a specific number of nursing staff per resident. This number must be on the floor at all times. Make sure there is a registered nurse present at each shift. Check to see how calls are handled on weekends.

- **Are Animals Allowed to Visit?** A visit from the family pet can do wonders for morale.

- **Items That May Be Brought from Home** Most facilities allow certain items to be brought from home. It helps to know what can be brought in advance of the move.

- **What Are the Visiting Hours?** Are family members welcomed anytime of the day?

- **Roommates** If there is a problem, how will it be handled, and by whom?

- **Diapers** Who orders the diapers, where are they stored, and who has access to that storage?

- **Laundry** How should clothing be marked?

- **Types of Clothing** Most sites recommend sweats and other loose fitting clothes. For women they recommend duster robes. House shoes or slipper socks work well and are not as slippery as shoes.

- **What Are the Extra Charges?** The homes handle the little extras in different ways. Visits to the Beauty or Barber Shop are usually charged extra. Find out about these charges.

    Some of these questions seem petty or, at least, picky. The only way to avoid misunderstanding is to have an understanding. Surprises after the fact are not any fun.

ADMISSION TO A NURSING HOME

Information Needed

Personal information:
Date of Birth
Place of Birth
Marital Status
Social Security Number/Card
Medicare Card
Medicaid Card
Insurance Policy Card
Ambulance Service

Medical Information:
Doctor's Orders Including:
    Medication
    Treatments
    Diet Orders
    Activity Level
If Doctor Will Follow Them in Nursing Home
Current History And Physical
Recent Lab Or X-rays
Discharge Summary From Last Hospitalization

Financial Information (For Planning Purposes):
List of Assets
List of Income
List of Liabilities

Other Information—Bring Copies of This Information:
Durable Power of Attorney For Health Care
Advanced Directives/Living Will
Legal Guardianship

MEDICAID INFORMATION

Information needed when going to the Department Of Human Services to apply for Medicaid.

1. Social Security Card
2. Insurance policies and the amount of each premium for hospital, medical, and life insurance
3. Proof of income
4. Legal description of any land, real estate, or mineral rights
5. Bank statements for all checking, savings, stock, and bonds
6. Papers relating to burial policies, trust, or contract with funeral home
7. Citizenship and alien permits if applicable
8. Medicare card
9. Doctor's name and address
10. Explanation of need
11. Proof of any transfer of property during the last five years along with all papers relating to such transfers

ALTERNATIVE METHODS OF FINANCING

Since both Reverse Mortgage and Viatical Settlements are relatively new methods for financing long-term care, I interviewed two people who sell these products. I also asked two attorneys for their opinions on the value of these approaches. Both attorneys saw merit in their use. Both suggested that families select established companies who understand these products. Both also suggested that the family get a second opinion from a financial planner or a CPA on the offers made by the companies.

Reverse Mortgage

I interviewed Audra Pickens who is with a company called The Reverse Mortgage Company in Norman, Oklahoma. Her company is connected with The Unity Mortgage Corp. Listing these names does not constitute an endorsement in any way. I am sure there are many great companies in this field.

Q What is a reverse mortgage?
A A reverse mortgage is a special kind of mortgage loan for seniors. It is a safe and easy way to turn your home equity into cash. Unlike a home equity loan, you do not have to make monthly payments. The reverse mortgage pays you and the loan is repaid when you no longer live in the house.

Q How does a person qualify?
A You must be 62 or older and either own or almost own your home.

Q How safe are these loans?
A These loans are backed by FHA and Fannie Mae. They guarantee you can stay in your home as long as you like, and you will never owe more than the home is worth.

Q What are the dangers?
A There are a lot of companies offering to refinance homes. These can be confused with reverse mortgages. A family should use caution in choosing a company that specializes in reverse mortgages. Remember a reverse mortgage pays you each month. With a home equity loan you pay them each month.

Viatical Settlements

I interviewed Tom Moran who is with a company called Viaticus. Viaticus is owned by C.N.A. Insurance.

Q I have never heard of Viatical Settlements. Is this a new thing?
A Viatical settlements grew out of an effort to help people suffering with AIDS. Most of these people were young and not eligible for Medicare. The idea was developed to allow people who were chronically or terminally ill to sell their insurance and use the money for their care.

Q How do people quality?
A There are several ways to qualify.
1. anyone who is diagnosed as chronic or terminally ill.
2. anyone over 65 who has health problems.
3. anyone over 70 who has even minor problems.
4. anyone over 75 can qualify with no health requirements.

Q Are these funds taxed?
A If the person is properly qualified, the funds are not taxed. This makes Viatical Settlements a very good tool for estate planning as well as long-term care.

Q Since this is new, how does a person find a company that sells this product?
A The Viatical Association of America is a national organization of reputable companies and agents. This organization maintains a toll free number, 1-800-842-9811.

Q What are the dangers in this product?
A A person should deal with a reputable company that is qualified to provide this settlement tax free. They should have their offer looked at by a disinterested third party. They should also inform the family of their intentions.

Long-Term Care Insurance

I interviewed Jane Moran who specializes in Long-Term Care Insurance. Since Jane is an independent agent she has access to the policies offered by several companies and spends a great deal of her time comparing these policies.

Q I am amazed at how few people in my seminars know about Long-Term Care Insurance, much less own a policy. Why is this such a secret?
A This coverage is relatively new. It took the insurance companies several years to understand what people needed and to design the coverage to meet these needs. It has taken some time for individual agents to become proficient in all of the various coverages and to get comfortable offering the policies to their clients.

Q I had to ask my agent about this coverage and he had to spend time studying the subject. I think I was his first sale. What is long-term care insurance?
A Long-Term Care Insurance provides the funds for care in those times when we need outside help for an extended period of time. It is wrong to think of it only as Nursing Home insurance. These policies can be written to cover assisted living and other types of facilities, and can also cover care in the home. Nor is this "Old Folks" insurance. Many younger people need care following accidents and illnesses that demand care beyond regular insurance. Statistics show we are more

likely to need this coverage than we are the coverage on our houses or cars.

Q **Is there an age at which a person is too old to purchase this care?**
A That depends on the person and the situation. I recently wrote a policy for an eighty-two year old lady. The older we are when we purchase this coverage, the more costly the coverage is, but when one compares the cost of long-term nursing care, it may still be a viable expenditure.

Q **There are so many variables in the coverage and so many policies on the market. How can I know what coverage to buy and what company to trust?**
A The best advice I can give is for families to find an insurance company that has a Long-Term Care Specialist on their staff. Since there are so many variables to explore they need someone who spends most of their time studying the coverage. The second bit of advice is that they find companies who are well established in this field. Those who have been involved long enough to study the needs and form their coverage to meet these needs.

Q **When I asked you to list the most important things to consider in purchasing this insurance, you sent me three pages of detailed information. We do not have room to print all of the information you felt we needed to know. If I contact a reputable company**

with a specialist in this area, are the chances good that I will get a policy that fits my needs?
A I think the chances are more than good. More agents and companies are specializing in this insurance. Good agents selling good products are now available in almost every area.

Other Elder Care Resources by Doug Manning from In-Sight Books:

When Love Gets Tough—Making the Nursing Home Decision

Parenting Our Parents

Searching for Normal Feelings

Visiting in a Nursing Home

Socks—How to Solve Problems

Caring for Elderly Loved Ones cassette

Planning The Care of Aging Loved Ones video series:
Family Issues
Legal and Financial Issues
Selection Issues
Guilt Issues
Caregiver Issues

In-Sight Books, Inc.
1-800-658-9262

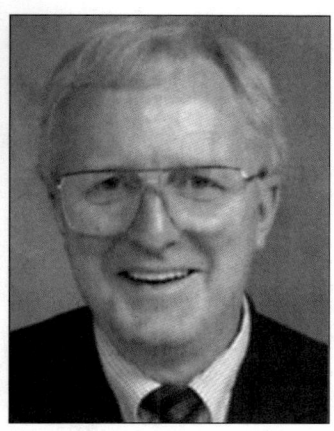

Doug Manning

Doug Manning is the author of twenty books designed to help people face the tough issues of life.

After thirty years as a minister and counselor, he began a new career almost twenty years ago as an author and speaker. Doug and his wife, Barbara, have been long-term caregivers to three parents.

Doug has a warm conversational style in which he shares his insights from his various experiences. Contact In-Sight Books at 1-800-658-9262 for a complete catalog of his products or visit our website at www.insightbooks.com.

ISBN 1-892785-27-7